THE GAPS DIET

COOKBOOK

FOR

NEWBIES AND BEGINNERS

BY

Dr. Christen Zimmermann

TABLE OF CONTENTS

The GAPS diet theory says that eliminating certain foods, such as grains and sugars, can help people treat conditions that affect the brain, such as autism and dyslexia.

What is the GAPS diet?

The term GAPS is an acronym for Gut and Psychology Syndrome; a condition recognized through years of clinical experience and observation by Neurologist, Dr Natasha Campbell-McBride, who identified a link between an individual's state of gut health and neurological or psychological health conditions such as obsessive compulsive disorder (OCD), attention deficit hyperactivity disorder (ADHD and ADD), autism, depression, anxiety and much more.

We now know that many common health conditions can be attributed to what is happening in the gut. This includes food intolerances, allergies, autoimmune diseases, weight issues (over and underweight), asthma, skin conditions such as eczema, acne, psoriasis, digestive disorders such as Crohn's, IBS, ulcerative colitis, and even heart conditions.

The GAPS diet is an intervention protocol that helps to detoxify the body, especially the digestive system, to enable healing of the gut lining and re-population of gut bacteria, improving gut health and overall health and wellbeing. Many people that follow the GAPS diet find that they are able to clear up many of the health complaints listed above.

There are two parts to the GAPS diet. The Introduction diet which has 6 stages and the Full GAPS diet. The protocol eliminates inflammatory and hard to digest foods, while maintaining and re-introducing nourishing foods. This allows the gut to heal while still providing nourishment to the body.

How to approach GAPS

One of the most important things to remember is that GAPS is not a one-size-fits-all approach. It is necessary to tailor the diet to suit the individual, depending on how severe your condition is. Some people can move through the first stage of the Introduction diet in a few days, perhaps spending more time in stage two. Others may need to stay on stage one for longer due to being unable to cope with many vegetables. Some can go through the 6 stages of the Introduction diet in three months, others may take a year or more.

For those with food intolerances and allergies, it is important to go through the Introduction phase very slowly and carefully, with the help of an experienced GAPS practitioner (who has personally been through GAPS, not just studied it). Food intolerances and allergies are a result of the gut lining being "leaky", which does not allow food to be digested and absorbed properly and provokes an immune reaction against undigested food particles. Healing and sealing the gut should clear up most, if not all food allergies and sensitivities.

Slow Cooker Beef Bone Broth Recipe

If you haven't heard about the benefits of bone broth, we're here to fill you in. Bone broth is made by simmering bones with water and vegetables for a long time, thereby extracting a host of benefits.

Ingredients

• 4 pounds mixed beef bones marrow bones, oxtail, knuckles, short rib, etc.

• 2 medium onions

• 2 medium carrots

• 3 stalks celery

• 1 bay leaf

• 2 tablespoons apple cider vinegar

Instructions

1. Heat oven to 400°F.

2. Spread the mixed bones on a baking tray in a single layer and place it into the oven. Roast the bones for 30 minutes. Flip bones and roast another 30 minutes.

3. While the bones are roasting, chop the carrots, onions and celery. (You are discarding these later so a rough chop works great!)

4. Place roasted bones, chopped vegetables, bay leaf and apple cider vinegar into a 6-Quart crockpot. Cover completely with cold filtered water. (All the ingredients should be submerged by about 1 inch of water.)

5. Cook on low for 24 hours. Add water as needed to keep all the ingredients covered in water, and periodically skim the foam off the top of the pot.

6. After 24 hours, the broth should be a dark brown color. Strain the broth through a fine mesh strainer and discard the bones, vegetables and bay leaf.

7. Before storing, pour into separate containers and cool to room temperature. Once cooled, chill in the refrigerator for 1-2 hours. Skim off the accumulated fat at the top of the container, if there's any. Store in the fridge for up to a week or in the freezer for up to 3 months.

This is a savory turkey bone broth you can make from the carcass of a roasted turkey. Make it in advance and store it to use in meals, soups, and stews.

Ingredients

• 1 turkey carcass from a roasted bird (it's OK to have some meat and skin attached to the bones)

• Turkey giblets

• 1 large onion, coarsely chopped

• 6 cloves garlic, smashed

• 1 cup parsley (1 small bunch)

• 1 mandarin orange peel (orange peel or lemon peel works too)

• 2 bay leaves

• 7 Quarts filtered water

Instructions

1. Place the turkey carcass and giblets in a large stockpot. Add the onion, garlic, parsley, orange peel, and bay leaves, and cover with cold water.

2. Bring to a boil and reduce the heat to medium-low. Simmer for 8-10 hours.

3. Discard the solids and strain the broth through a fine-mesh strainer into a large container. Ladle the broth into mason jars. Once it's cool, you'll be able to remove the fat on the surface easily with a spoon. Enjoy and refrigerate or freeze the leftovers for later.

Pork Broth

Pork broth has its own unique flavor and can serve as a base for a number of Asian dishes, including soups, stews, and stir fries. A homemade batch of pork broth can last in your refrigerator for a week or so (or you can freeze it for longer) and can add flavor to rice or sauteed vegetables, or even braise a larger cut of pork.

Ingredients:

• 2 pounds pork bones (ideally feet, neck, and/or rib bones)

• 1 yellow onion, coarsely chopped

• 4 ribs celery, coarsely chopped

• 1 head garlic, smashed to release flavor (no need to peel)

• 3 tablespoons apple cider vinegar

• Filtered water, filled 2-3 inches from the top of the pot

• 2 teaspoons sea salt

Optional ingredients for a Thai flavor:

• 4 scallions, chopped (instead of the yellow onion)

• 2 inches fresh ginger, chopped

• 1 stalk fresh lemongrass, outer layer removed and coarsely chopped

• 1 large daikon radish, chopped

Directions:

1. Rinse the pork bones and add to the pot.

2. Add apple cider vinegar and fill with cold water.

3. Let sit for at least 30 minutes before turning on the heat.

4. Add all other ingredients and turn up the stove to high heat for 20 minutes.

5. Once the liquid is at a roiling boil, turn to low heat.

6. Allow to simmer partially covered for 6 to 24 hours, skimming the top with the mesh strainer a few times throughout the process to remove any foam or scum that rises to the top.

7. When finished, strain broth into jars or containers. Allow the broth to cool to room temperature before refrigerating or freezing for later use.

This is a Kettle & Fire tested and true slow cooker chicken bone broth recipe that features organic chicken bones, fresh vegetables, and herbs.

Ingredients

• 2 pounds chicken bones leftover from roasted chicken, preferably organic

• 2 stalks celery roughly chopped

• 2 carrots skin on, roughly chopped

• 1 yellow or white onion roughly chopped

• 1 green bell pepper roughly chopped

• 1 head garlic

• 1/2 cup fresh parsley

• 1/4 cup fresh thyme

• 2 sprigs rosemary

• 2 bay leaves

• 1 tablespoon whole peppercorns

• 8-10 cups filtered water or enough to cover ingredients

Instructions

1. Rinse vegetables and herbs and place into a slow cooker.

2. Add chicken bones and all remaining ingredients to slow cooker and cover with enough water so that all ingredients are submerged.

3. Turn on slow cooker to low heat and let cook for 12-18 hours.

4. Remove from heat and carefully separate the vegetables and bones from the broth.

5. Strain the broth into a bowl through a colander, and strain once more through a cheesecloth to remove any remaining particles.

6. Pour broth into an airtight jar and store in the refrigerator for up to a week, or freeze for up to 3 months.

Homemade SCD GAPS Diet Yogurt

This Homemade SCD GAPS Diet Yogurt is fermented for 24 hours, making it virtually lactose free and easier to digest. Enjoy with fresh fruit and honey for breakfast for an afternoon snack.

Ingredients

• 1/2 gallon grass-fed organic whole milk

• 1/2 cup plain yogurt containing Lactobacillus bulgaricus L. acidophilus and S. thermophilus

Instructions

1. Heat milk in a large pot until it reaches a simmer, about 180 degrees fahrenheit.

2. Let cool to room temperature (I let it cool down to 80 degrees).

3. Remove 1 cup of cooled milk to a bowl and stir in yogurt until blended. Stir into pot and mix until blended. Divide milk among mason jars.

4. Place in dehydrator and set to 105 degrees fahrenheit. Leave undisturbed for 24 hours. Remove and set in refrigerator until ready to eat.

5. Eat within 2 weeks.

Creamy Tomato Soup with Coconut and Curry

Coconut milk, bone broth, and a hint of turmeric-tinted curry make this creamy tomato soup a wholesome, dairy-free version of the classic that's sure to become one of your new favorite homemade tomato soup recipes.

Ingredients

- 2 tablespoons coconut oil

- 1 red onion chopped

- 1 red bell pepper chopped

- 1 carrot chopped

- Kosher salt

- 1 clove garlic minced

- 24 ounces canned whole peeled tomatoes

- 2 teaspoons curry powder

- 1.5 cups Kettle & Fire Chicken Bone Broth

- 1 cup canned full-fat coconut milk

- 1 lime cut into quarters

• Freshly ground black pepper

• Optional garnish: Microgreens and hemp seeds

Instructions

1. In a medium pot over medium-high heat, warm the coconut oil until melted. Add the onion, bell pepper, carrot, and a pinch of salt and cook, stirring occasionally, until the vegetables are soft, 4 to 6 minutes.

2. Add the garlic and curry powder and cook until fragrant, about 1 minute. Then stir in the tomatoes and a pinch of salt. Cook, stirring, for another minute. Add the broth and simmer until the tomatoes are cooked, 10 to 15 minutes. Remove from the heat and blend until smooth with an immersion blender or regular blender.

3. Return to the stove over medium heat. Stir in the coconut milk and a squeeze of lime and cook for another minute. Season with salt and pepper to taste. Garnish with microgreens and hemp seeds, if using.

Butternut S☐uash Soup

Butternut s☐uash soup is a rich, creamy comfort food that's often loaded with milk or heavy cream and butter. Our version of this tasty treat uses full-fat coconut milk and ghee instead, giving you the same rich experience without the lactose that may bother those with gut issues.) and sugars.

Ingredients

• 1 large butternut s☐uash

• 2 tablespoons ghee or coconut oil

• ½ large yellow onion chopped

• 2 cloves garlic chopped

• 1.5- inch piece fresh ginger chopped

• 2 cups Kettle & Fire Chicken Bone Broth

• 1 teaspoon sea salt plus more to taste

• ¼ teaspoon sumac

• ¼ teaspoon red chili flake

• ½ teaspoon cinnamon

- 1 cup water

- ¾ cup canned coconut milk

- 1 teaspoon apple cider vinegar

- OPTIONAL TOPPING: freshly ground black pepper extra virgin olive oil, fresh sage, and avocado oil for frying

Instructions

1. Place whole squash in a shallow baking pan and bake at 425°F for 1 hour 20 minutes, turning half-way through. When the squash is ready (it will give when you press on the skin), remove from the oven and cut in half. Scoop out the seeds, remove skin, and discard. Cut the roasted squash into 2-inch cubes.

2. While the squash is baking, loosely chop the yellow onion and garlic.

3. In a large stock pot over medium heat, melt the ghee. Add the onions and cook until translucent, about 5 minutes. Add the garlic and ginger, stirring to make sure the garlic doesn't burn. Stir in the squash and cook until combined, 3 minutes.

4. Stir in the bone broth, salt, sumac, red chili and cinnamon. Cover and cook for another 10 minutes. Remove from the heat.

5. Transfer the soup to a blender and blend until smooth. (Optionally, leave half of the soup unblended for a chunkier soup).

6. Return the blended soup to the pot. Turn the heat to low, then stir in water, coconut milk, and apple cider vinegar. Cook for another minute or two until warmed through. Add salt and black pepper, to taste. Serve.

Sweet Potato Toast

This is one of the easiest and most satisfying comfort food breakfasts you'll ever have — especially if you're an egg and avocado toast fan. But rather than using traditional whole grain bread, this recipe calls for oven-roasted sweet potatoes, which makes it Whole30 Plan approved and paleo friendly.

Ingredients

• 1 large sweet potato

• ½ tablespoon extra virgin olive oil

• 4 large eggs

• 1 avocado

• ¼ teaspoon garlic salt

• ¼ teaspoon crushed red pepper chili flakes

Instructions

1. Heat the oven to 375°F.

2. While the oven is heating, cut sweet potato into four quarter-inch thick slices with a very sharp knife.

3. Line a baking sheet with parchment paper and place the four sweet potato slices on the paper. Drizzle olive oil over the sweet potatoes to evenly coat. Transfer to the oven and bake for 20 minutes, or until soft and slightly browned.

4. While the sweet potatoes are baking, bring 6 cups of water to a boil in a medium-sized pot. Once the water is boiling, carefully place eggs into the pot and let boil for exactly 6 minutes.

5. Slice the avocado in half and spoon into a small bowl, discarding the pit. Add the garlic, sea salt and smash lightly with a fork.

6. Once the eggs are done, carefully peel the shell under cold running water.

7. Assemble on a plate using the sweet potato as the toast. Spread avocado mash onto the toast, top with soft-boiled eggs, and garnish with crushed red pepper chili flakes.

Paleo Pumpkin Soup with Bone Broth and Coconut Milk

Curling up with a bowl of this comforting, creamy, spiced pumpkin soup makes heading into the colder months much easier.

Ingredients

• 1 cup Kettle & Fire Chicken Bone Broth

• ½ cup coconut milk

• 1 can pure pumpkin

• ½ teaspoon ground ginger

• ½ teaspoon paprika

• ½ teaspoon ground nutmeg

• ½ teaspoon garlic powder

• ½ teaspoon cinnamon

• ½ teaspoon sea salt

• ½ teaspoon ground black pepper

• 1 tablespoon sour cream optional

• 1 tablespoon pumpkin seeds roasted (optional)

Instructions

1. In a large pot over medium heat, add chicken bone broth, coconut milk, pumpkin and spices.

2. Bring to a boil, then reduce the heat and let simmer for 10 minutes, stirring occasionally.

3. Serve in small bowls. Garnish with sour cream and pumpkin seeds.

The Best Cast Iron Skillet Chicken Soup

The tender, juicy chicken breast in this soup is flavored with herbs and aromatics, including parsley, garlic, onion and black pepper. The addition of savory chicken bone broth guarantees the flavor factor.

Ingredients

• 2 bone-in skin-on chicken thighs

• ¼ teaspoon sea salt

• ¼ teaspoon ground black pepper

• 1 tablespoon grass-fed butter

• 2 cloves garlic minced

• ½ onion finely chopped

• 2 cups Kettle & Fire Chicken Bone Broth

• ½ cup frozen peas thawed

• 1 tablespoon chopped parsley

Instructions

1. Heat the oven to 425°F.

2. Using a paper towel, pat both sides of the chicken thighs dry and rub salt and pepper onto the chicken.

3. In a large skillet over medium heat, melt the butter. Place the chicken thighs skin-side down on the skillet. Cook for 5 minutes. Flip and cook for 2 more minutes.

4. Divide garlic, onion, chicken bone broth and peas evenly between two small cast iron skillets.

5. Add one chicken thigh to each skillet and place in the oven for 30 minutes, or until chicken is fully cooked.

6. Serve chicken soup in the cast iron skillet and garnish with parsley.

Slow Cooker Pot Roast With Beef Bone Broth

A tender beef slow cooker pot roast, cooked in beef bone broth for extra flavour and simmered with rosemary and thyme. Served with sweet potatoes, this hassle-free recipe is what Sunday dinner dreams are made of.

Ingredients

• 3 pounds chuck roast

• 6 carrots roughly chopped

• 2 sweet potatoes cut into ½-inch cubes

• 2 onions halved

• 2 sprigs fresh rosemary

• 3 sprigs fresh thyme

• ½ teaspoon Kosher salt

• ½ teaspoon ground black pepper

Instructions

1. In a large crock pot, add all of the ingredients.

2. Cook on high heat for 4 hours. (Or 8 hours on low heat).

3. Remove herb stems and enjoy.

Creamy Asparagus Soup with Avocado and Fennel

Asparagus season is almost in full swing, and there's no better way to eat it than in a creamy soup form. This velvety asparagus soup has all the best ⓠualities of a traditional velouté without any of the added flour or heavy cream.

Ingredients

• 2 tablespoons olive oil plus more for serving

• 1 large leek white and pale green parts finely chopped

• 1 bulb fennel thinly sliced

• Kosher salt

• 4 cups Kettle & Fire Chicken Bone Broth

• 2 pounds asparagus trimmed and cut into 1-inch pieces

• 1 tablespoon lemon thyme leaves minced

• 1 lemon juiced

• 1 avocado peeled, pitted, and diced

• Freshly ground black pepper

• Greek yogurt for serving (optional)

Instructions

1. In a large saucepan over medium-low heat, warm oil. Add leek and fennel and a large pinch of salt. Cook, stirring frequently, until fully softened but not browned, 3 to 5 minutes. Stir in bone broth and bring to a simmer.

2. Add asparagus and thyme. Bring to a simmer and cook for 1 minute. Remove a few asparagus tips and use them for garnish. Continue simmering soup until asparagus is soft, 4 to 5 minutes. Remove from heat and add lemon juice and avocado.

3. Blend soup using an immersion blender or in batches using a blender until it's smooth. Season to taste with salt and pepper and serve. Garnish with reserved asparagus tips, fennel fronds, olive oil and greek yogurt, if using.

Green Bone Broth Smoothie

Bone broth is a versatile ingredient that can enhance a variety of recipes. This delicious smoothie stars Kettle & Fire Beef Bone Broth made from the bones of 100% grass-fed cattle.

Ingredients

• 3-4 Kettle & Fire Beef Bone Broth ice cubes

• 1 cup spinach rinsed

• 1 banana peeled and sliced

• 1 green apple cored and sliced

• 1/2 cup water

Instructions

1. Make bone broth ice cubes the night prior by pouring Kettle and Fire Beef Bone Broth into ice tray.

2. Place the spinach, banana, and apple in a blender with ½ cup of water. Add 3-4 beef bone broth ice cubes.

3. Blend on high speed for 30-45 seconds or until smooth. Pour into a glass and enjoy!

Beef Ragu with Spaghetti Squash

This dish harkens back to the old country with traditional Italian herbs, a rich tomato base, and grass-fed ground beef. Sink your teeth into our pasta substitute, a sweet and savory spaghetti squash that you can twirl on your fork just like the real thing.

Ingredients

• 1 medium spaghetti squash

• 2 tablespoons ghee

• 1 pound grass-fed ground beef

• 1 leek chopped from root to tip

• 2 teaspoons extra virgin olive oil

• 2 sprigs rosemary leaves minced

• 2 sprigs parsley leaves minced

• 2 sprigs oregano leaves minced

• 2 sprigs sage leaves minced

• ½ cup Kettle & Fire Beef Bone Broth

• 3 cups canned tomatoes strained

• 1 teaspoon raw apple cider vinegar

• Salt and pepper

• 2 tablespoons parmesan cheese optional

Instructions

1. Set the oven to broil and place the whole spaghetti squash on a baking pan. Transfer to the oven, and broil for 15 minutes on one side. Then turn over and broil for another 15 minutes. You'll know it's done when it gives a bit to pressure. Remove the spaghetti squash from the oven and cut in half, taking care that the steam doesn't burn your hands.

2. While the squash is cooking, make the sauce. In a large sauce pan over medium heat, warm 1 tablespoon of ghee. Add ground beef and cook until just brown. Remove meat from pan and set aside.

3. Add 2 teaspoons extra virgin olive oil and the chopped leek to the pan and cook, stirring, until tender, about 3 minutes.

4. Add the meat back to the pan. Stir in half the herbs, bone broth, and strained tomatoes. Turn the heat to a

simmer and cook for another 15 minutes. Then add apple cider vinegar and a generous pinch of salt and pepper to the sauce and stir to combine. Remove from the heat.

5. When the squash is cool enough to handle, remove the seeds and sprinkle a pinch of salt into each half. Fluff with a fork to remove the stringy part of the squash. Divide evenly into four large dinner bowls to create the "spaghetti."

6. Top each bowl of squash with about 1 cup of sauce and the remaining fresh herbs. Finish with cheese, if using.

Keto Meatloaf

A juicy, flavor-packed keto meatloaf topped with a tangy and sweet tomato sauce that is gluten-free and low carb to meet your keto diet needs.

Ingredients

For the meatloaf:

• 1 ½ pounds ground beef

• 2 large cage-free eggs

• 1 small onion diced

• 2 cloves garlic minced

• 2 cups mushrooms finely chopped

• 1 teaspoon coconut aminos

• 1 tablespoon tomato paste

• ¼ cup unsweetened almond milk

• ¼ cup almond flour

• 1 tablespoon dried oregano

• 1 teaspoon Himalayan pink salt

- 1 teaspoon ground black pepper

For the tomato sauce:

- 1 cup tomatoes diced

- ½ teaspoon Himalayan pink salt

- ½ teaspoon ground black pepper

- ½ teaspoon dried oregano

- ½ teaspoon dried parsley

- 1 heirloom tomato sliced, (optional)

Instructions

1. Heat oven to 350°F.

2. In a large bowl, combine all the meatloaf ingredients and knead the mixture with your hands until fully combined.

3. In a non-stick, 9x5-inch loaf pan, add the meatloaf mixture and press down to fill all the edges of the pan. Set aside.

4. In a small pot over low heat, add the tomato sauce ingredients and bring to a simmer. Cook for 2 minutes, stirring occasionally. Remove from the heat.

5. Pour the tomato sauce over the meatloaf. (If using, add slices of heirloom tomato to garnish). Place in the oven and cook until the meatloaf is cooked through and no longer pink in the middle, about 50 minutes.

6. Remove from the oven and let rest until warm, about 10 minutes. Serve.

Mixed Berry Bone Broth Smoothie

Blend and enjoy this mixed berry bone broth smoothie, a fruity treat for your body!

This bone broth smoothie recipe combines the broth with the strong flavors of fruit, so you'll barely notice it's there. To get a great bone broth smoothie texture and coldness, we suggest you make bone broth ice cubes the night before making your smoothie. Simply pour Kettle and Fire chicken bone broth into an ice cube tray and freeze it.

Ingredients

• 3-4 Kettle & Fire Chicken Bone Broth ice cubes

• 1 cup mixed berries, rinsed

• 1 banana, peeled and sliced

• ¼ cup flaxseeds

• ½ cup water

Instructions

1. Make bone broth ice cubes the night prior by pouring Kettle and Fire Chicken Bone Broth into an ice tray and freeze it.

2. Place the mixed berries, banana, and flax seeds in a blender with ½ cup of water. Add 3-4 chicken bone broth ice cubes. Blend until smooth.

3. Pour into a glass and enjoy!

Chicken Parmesan with Zucchini Noodles (Grain Free, Paleo, Gluten Free)

Chicken Parmesan is a classic dish and I've upgraded the ingredients so they are all grain-free!

Ingredients

For the Noodles:

• 2 pounds zucchini, cut into noodles using a noodle slicer

• 1/2 teaspoon Celtic sea salt

For the Chicken:

• 4 boneless skinless chicken breasts, pounded

• Celtic sea salt

• 1 cup almond flour (if you are allergic to nuts, then use 1/3 arrowroot flour, 1/3 tapioca flour and 1/3 coconut flour)

• 2 large eggs, beaten

• 2 tablespoons ghee

• 1/2 cup grated Pecorino Romano or Mozzarella (omit if Paleo) (I use Pecorino Romano in place of Parmesan because it's more economical and has a nice salty bite.)

For the Spaghetti Sauce:

• 1 tablespoon extra-virgin olive oil

• 2 cloves garlic, minced

• 1 (24-ounce) jar crushed tomatoes

• 1/2 teaspoon Celtic sea salt

• 1/2 teaspoon dried Italian seasoning

Instructions

1. Place zucchini noodles in a colander and season with salt. Toss. Let sit for 20 minutes. Place a clean dish towel on the counter and pour zucchini on to towel. Fold towel over zucchini and gently press to dry noodles.

2. Preheat broiler to high. Season chicken with sea salt. Place flour in one flat-bottom dish and the eggs in another. Heat large skillet over medium heat for 2 minutes. Add ghee, melt, and swirl to coat. Dip chicken into the eggs, then the almond flour and place into the

pan. Repeat with remaining chicken pieces. Cook, without moving, for 4 minutes until bottom is golden brown. Flip chicken and cook another 4-5 minutes until second side is golden brown. Remove and place on a cooling rack set over a large baking sheet (this keeps the crust from getting soggy). Place a piece of mozzarella (or some shredded Pecorino Romano) on each piece of chicken. Broil until melted.

3. Meanwhile, heat olive oil and garlic in a medium saucepan over medium heat. When garlic begins to sizzle, add tomatoes, salt and Italian seasoning (try to stand back a bit, as the sauce may splatter). Simmer on low for 10 minutes.

4. Wipe now-empty skillet with paper towels and pour 2 tablespoons olive oil in pan and heat over medium heat. Add zucchini noodles and using a pair of tongs, toss, until hot, about 2 minutes.

5. Serve chicken with marinara and zucchini noodles.

Butternut Squash Soup

Butternut S⍰uash Soup is a fall and winter favorite that's loaded with nourishing ingredients!

Ingredients

- 4 tablespoons ghee, divided
- 4 shallots, chopped
- 1 large butternut s⍰uash, peeled and cut into large bite-size pieces
- 1/2 teaspoon Celtic sea salt plus more for seasoning
- 1 teaspoon dried thyme
- 6 cups chicken stock
- 1/2 cup coconut milk

Instructions

1. Preheat oven to 400°F and adjust rack to middle position. Place 2 tablespoons ghee in a large pot over medium heat. Add shallots and stir. Reduce heat to low, cover pot with a lid and cook for 20 minutes.

2. Toss butternut squash with remaining 2 tablespoons melted ghee and spread evenly on a large baking dish. Season with sea salt. Roast for 15 minutes. Using a spatula, flip the butternut pieces and then roast for an additional 15 minutes, or until the squash is golden brown on the outside and soft on the inside.

3. Stir dried thyme into shallot mixture until fragrant, about 30 seconds. Pour in stock and add butternut squash. Bring to a simmer and cook for 15 minutes. Using a hand-immersion blender, blend soup until smooth (or you can spoon the soup into a blender and blend until smooth). Stir in coconut milk and season with sea salt. Serve.

Roast Beef Tenderloin

Roast Beef Tenderloin makes an appearance at only those truly special occasions. It's not a cheap dinner, so it's incredibly important you cook it correctly. We want to end up with a moist, juicy, tender piece of meat.

Ingredients

• 1 4-5 pound beef tenderloin, trimmed (if you'd like a small roast and one that's pastured, I highly recommend this one)

• 1 cup fermented tamari or coconut aminos

• 1/4 cup red wine vinegar

• 2 tablespoons ground garlic

• ?1 tablespoon freshly ground black pepper

• 2 tablespoons ghee , tallow ,or lard

Instructions

1. Place the tenderloin in a shallow baking dish. Stir together tamari and vinegar and pour over the roast. Season the meat with all the garlic and black pepper.

Marinate for 4 hours, rotating after 2 hours. Let the roast sit at room temperature for 1 hour before cooking.

2. Preheat the oven to 425°F and adjust the rack to the middle position. Place a large skillet over medium-high heat for 2 minutes. Add the ghee and swirl the pan to coat. Place the roast on the skillet and cook for 3-4 minutes until bottom is turning golden brown. Using a pair of tongs, turn the meat and cook for another 3-4 minutes until golden brown. Repeat this until all 4 sides are seared.

3. Transfer the roast to a large baking sheet, insert the thermometer in the thickest part of the roast and place in the oven. Roast for about 25-35 minutes, until thermometer reads 125°F for medium-rare. Remove from the oven and let the meat rest for 10 minutes before serving.

Roasted Butternut Squash with Goat Cheese and Pecans

Roasted butternut squash with goat cheese and pecans is a wonderful vegetarian side dish for a weeknight dinner or holiday meal.

Ingredients

• 1 2-3 pound butternut squash, skin and seeds removed and cut into 1/2" thick slices

• 3 tablespoons ghee , melted

• 1/2 teaspoon Celtic sea salt

• 1/8 teaspoon cayenne

• 1/4 cup goat cheese, crumbled

• 1/2 cup pecans, toasted and chopped

• 1 teaspoon fresh thyme leaves

Instructions

1. Preheat the oven to 425°F and adjust the rack to the lowest position. Place the squash in a large bowl and toss with the ghee, sea salt and cayenne. Spread the squash in an even layer on a baking sheet lined with parchment

paper. Roast for 25-30 minutes until well browned. Remove the squash from the oven and, using a pair of tongs, flip each piece of squash. Then, continue to roast in the oven until the face-down side of the s◻uash is browned, about 10 more minutes.

2. Transfer the s◻uash to a platter and top with the goat cheese, pecans and fresh thyme. Serve warm.

Roasted Salmon with Chimichurri (Grain-Free, Paleo)

Roasted salmon with Chimichurri is an easy weeknight recipe. The chimichurri can be made days ahead of time and stored in the fridge. And, the sauce also tastes amazing over roasted or sautéed vegetables.

Ingredients

For the salmon:

• 4 skin-on wild salmon fillets

• Celtic Sea salt

For the Chimichurri:

• 1 cup fresh flat-leaf parsley leaves

• 1 cup fresh cilantro

• 3 cloves garlic

• 1/2 cup extra virgin olive oil

• 1/4 cup red wine vinegar

• 1 teaspoon Celtic Sea salt

Instructions

1. Preheat the oven to 400°F and adjust the rack to the middle position. Place the salmon on a baking dish lined with parchment paper. Sprinkle with Celtic Sea salt. Place the salmon in the oven and roast for 11 minutes.

2. Meanwhile, place the parsley, cilantro, garlic, and sea salt in a food processor and pulse until coarsely chopped, about 5 one-second pulses. Add the olive oil and vinegar and pulse, until combined, about 5 one-second pulses. Transfer to bowl; set aside.

3. Spoon the chimichurri over top of each salmon fillet and serve.

Lemon-Thyme Chicken Thighs (Grain-Free, Paleo)

This easy lemon thyme chicken thighs recipe is perfect for a weeknight dinner! The lemon, garlic and herbs are stuffed underneath the skin and then the chicken is rubbed with ghee and roasted until crispy.

Ingredients

• Zest from 1 lemon

• 1 tablespoon fresh lemon juice

• 2 cloves garlic, minced

• 1 tablespoon chopped cilantro

• 1 tablespoon chopped thyme

• 1/2 teaspoon Celtic Sea salt

• 4 bone-in, skin-on organic chicken thighs

• 2 tablespoons ghee , melted (or duck fat for dairy-free)

Instructions

1. Preheat the oven to 425°F and adjust the rack to the middle position. Place a wire cooling rack over a baking sheet.

2. Combine the lemon zest, juice, garlic, cilantro, thyme, and sea salt in a small bowl and stir to combine. Loosen the skin on the chicken things and insert about 1 tablespoon of lemon mixture under skin of each.

3. Brush each chicken thigh (bottom and top of thigh) with ghee and place on the wire rack.

4. Roast the chicken until the skin is golden brown and crisp and a thermometer inserted into the thickest part of the chicken, but not touching the bone registers 165°F, about 20-25 minutes. Remove the chicken from the oven and let it rest for 5 minutes. Serve

Tortilla Soup Recipe

For many years, Tortilla Soup has been a family favorite. The soup is cooked all in one pot and can put on the table in just 45 minutes!

Ingredients

For the soup:

• 5 cloves garlic, crushed with skins on

• 6 springs fresh oregano

• 6 sprigs of cilantro, plus 1/2 cup roughly chopped

• 8 cups chicken stock

• 2 pounds bone-in chicken breasts or 1 small 3-4 pound chicken

For the Toppings:

• 3 cups Siete tortilla chips

• 1 avocado, cubed

• 2 tomatoes, cut into bite-size chunks

• 1 lime, cut into quarters

• 1/2 cup sour cream (omit for Paleo and Gaps)

• 1/2 cup shredded cheddar cheese (omit for Paleo)

Instructions

1. Place the garlic cloves in a large dutch oven over medium-high heat. Cook, stirring frequently until garlic begins to darken, about 2-2 1/2 minutes. Remove the pot from the heat and let it cool for about 30 seconds and then add the chicken stock, oregano, cilantro, and chicken to the garlic. Place pot back on heat and bring to a boil and then reduce to a simmer. Simmer for about 30 minutes. When chicken is cooked through, remove the chicken from the broth mixture and set aside. With slotted spoon, strain out the rest of the garlic and herbs. Shred the chicken with a fork and then add back to the soup. Add salt and pepper if needed.

2. To serve, crumble a handful of tortilla chips into individual bowls and then ladle the broth over. Serve with cilantro, avocado, tomatoes, lime, cheese, and sour cream.

Salmon and Baby Greens Salad with Creamy Garlic Dressing

A good salmon salad is one of my favorite go-tos during the week. You can make the pickled red onions, the garlic yogurt dressing, and even cook the salmon ahead of time and store them in the fridge for the salad later.

Ingredients

For the onions:

• 1 red onion, sliced thin

• 1/2 cup white wine vinegar

• 1/2 cup apple cider vinegar

• 1/2 teaspoon raw honey

• 1/4 teaspoon Celtic sea salt

For the salmon:

• 12 ounces wild salmon fillet, cut into 4 pieces

• Celtic sea salt

• Freshly ground black pepper

For the salad:

• 8 ounces baby lettuces

• 1/2 English cucumber, sliced

• 1/4 cup capers

• 1/4 cup sprouted pumpkin seeds

• 1/2 pint cherry tomatoes, each cut in half

For the dressing:

• 1/3-3/4 cup garlic-yogurt dressing (depending on how saturated you like your salad to be)

Instructions

1. Place the red onion, vinegars, honey and sea salt in a mason jar. Screw the lid on and shake until combined. Unscrew the lid and, using a spoon, press down the onions so they are all submerged in the liquid. Set aside for at least 30 minutes. (Can be made 1-6 days ahead of time and stored in the refrigerator.)

2. Preheat the oven to 450°F and adjust the rack to the middle position. Season the salmon with sea salt and pepper. Place the salmon, skin down, on a baking sheet

lined with unbleached parchment paper. Roast, 12 minutes, until salmon is cooked through.

3. To assemble the salad, place the lettuces, cucumber, capers, pumpkin seeds, cherry tomatoes and 1/2 cup of pickled onions in a large salad bowl. Pour the dressing over top and toss. Using salad tongs, divide the salad onto four plates. Top with salmon and serve.

Braised Chicken Thighs with Squash and Kale (Grain-Free)

Braised Chicken is a comforting dish to make during the winter months. Other dishes I love to prepare in the winter are Lentil Soup with Swiss Chard and Sausage, Butter Chicken (always a hit!), and White Beans and Sausage in the Crock Pot.

Ingredients

• 4 pounds skin-on, bone-in chicken thighs (about 12), patted dry

• Celtic sea salt

• Freshly ground pepper

• 2 tablespoons ghee

• 1 bunch scallions, sliced into 1-inch pieces

• 1 dried chiles de árbol

• 2 tablespoons chopped ginger

• 3 cups chicken broth, divided

• 1/2 cup fermented gluten-free tamari or coconut aminos

- 2 tablespoons coconut sugar (or raw honey for GAPS)

- 2 tablespoons sesame oil

- 1 butternut squash, cut into bite-size pieces

- 1 bunch kale, chopped and steamed (this is why I prefer to cook the greens first, but if you'd like to add them raw, that will work as well)

- 1 tablespoon coconut vinegar

- 2 teaspoons toasted sesame seeds

Instructions

1. Lightly season the chicken thighs with sea salt and pepper. Heat the ghee in a large Dutch oven or other heavy pot over medium-high. Working in 2 batches, cook chicken, skin side down, until skin is browned and crisp, about 8–10 minutes. Transfer the chicken to a plate, placing skin side up (the chicken will not be cooked through at this point).

2. Keep the heat at medium-high (keep any leftover ghee, chicken fat, etc. in the pot) and place the scallions, chiles,

and ginger in the pot to cook, stirring frequently until onions are just turning golden brown on the edges, about 3 minutes.

3. Add 1 cup of chicken broth , bring to a simmer, and cook until reduced to about 3 tablespoons. This will take about 5 minutes. Add the tamari, coconut sugar, sesame oil, and remaining broth and bring to a simmer, stirring to dissolve sugar. Place the butternut squash and kale in the pot. Place the chicken, skin-side up on top of the squash and kale, and, using a pair of tongs, nestle each piece of chicken down into the liquid mixture so the bottom of each piece of chicken is in the liquid. Partially cover the pot, reduce the heat to medium-low, and simmer until the chicken and squash are cooked through, about 20 minutes.

4. Remove the chicken, increase the heat to medium, and continue to cook until liquid is reduced by about two-thirds and has the consistency of thin gravy, about 10–15 minutes.

5. Remove the pot from heat and drizzle the vinegar over the squash and kale mixture. Add the chicken back to pot,

turning to coat in sauce, and sprinkle sesame seeds over top.

6. This recipe can be made 2 days ahead. Let cool; cover and chill and then reheat covered over low heat.

Beef Stew (Grain Free, Gluten Free, Gaps, Paleo)

Beef stew is a comforting and nourishing meal that has become a family favorite. It's a great meal for an informal dinner since you can prepare it two days in advance and keep it in the refrigerator until you reheat it on the stove for your guests. A hearty salad provides a great complement and a bowl of chocolate mousse makes for a sweet ending.

Ingredients

• 2 tablespoons ghee , divided

• 4 yellow onions, sliced thin

• 2 tablespoons coconut flour

• 2 cloves garlic, minced

• 1 teaspoon dried thyme

• 1 1/2 cups dry white wine (you can substitute this with chicken stock)

• 1 1/2 cups chicken stock

• 3 pounds beef chuck, trimmed and cut into 1 1/2-inch pieces

• 1 tablespoon honey

• 1 tablespoon cider vinegar

• 2 bay leaves

• 2 teaspoons Celtic sea salt

• 1 tablespoon Dijon mustard

• 1/4 cup chopped flat-leaf parsley

Instructions

1. Preheat the oven to 250°F and place rack on middle-low position. Heat 2 tablespoons ghee in a large dutch oven (an ovenproof pot with a lid) over medium-low heat. Add the add onions and sauté, stirring frequently until onions release their liquid, about 10 minutes. (If the bottom of the pot begins to brown too much, push the onions aside with a spoon, pour a small amount of water and scrape up the brown bits.) Continue to cook until the onions caramelize, about 15 minutes. Stir in coconut flour and cook for 1 minute. Make a well in the center of the pot and add garlic and thyme and cook until fragrant, about 45 seconds. Add the wine and chicken stock, scraping up any brown bits on the bottom of the pan. Add the beef,

honey, cider vinegar, bay leaves and sea salt. Bring to a boil, cover with the lid and place in the oven. Cook for 2 1/2 hours, until meat is tender. Stir in mustard and parsley and additional sea salt to taste. Serve alone or over creamy mashed potatoes.

White Bean and Ham Soup Recipe

Fall is here, which means it's time for nourishing soups! This white bean soup with ham is warm and comforting, and best of all, it's completely prepared in a slow cooker.

Ingredients

For the Beans:

• 1 pound dried white navy beans

• Pinch of baking soda

For the Soup:

• 2 meaty smoked ham hocks (pastured preferred)

• 8 cups chicken stock

• 6 ribs celery, cut into bite-size pieces

• 6 carrots, cut into 1/2"-thick coins

• 1 yellow onion, chopped

• 10 cloves garlic, peeled and smashed

• 6 sprigs fresh thyme

• 2 teaspoons Celtic sea salt

Instructions

1. The night before, place the white beans in a large bowl and cover with water. Stir in a pinch of baking soda.

2. The next day, drain and rinse the beans and then place them in a slow cooker . Add the ham hocks, chicken stock, celery, carrots, onion, garlic, and thyme in the slow cooker and stir to combine. Cover and cook for about 6 hours on low until the beans are tender.

3. Using a pair of tongs, remove the thyme and ham hocks. Shred the ham and return it back to the slow cooker. Stir in the salt, taste and add more if needed. Serve.

Easy Slow Cooker Pepper Steak (Grain-Free, Paleo)

The end of the school year can be almost as busy as the holiday season, so it's a great time to pull out the slow cooker! One of our recent favorites is slow cooker pepper steak because it barely takes any time to prepare and at the end of the day the meat is melt-in-your-mouth tender and full of flavor.

Ingredients

• 2 red onions, peeled and cut into wedges

• 1 1/2 pounds chuck roast, cut into bite-size pieces

• 3 red, orange or yellow bell peppers, cut into wedges

• 1 cup chicken broth

• 1/4 cup coconut aminos or gluten-free fermented Tamari

• 1/4 cup tomato paste

• 4 garlic cloves, minced

Instructions

1. Place the onions in the bottom of the slow cooker. Top the onions with the meat and then add the bell peppers. Whisk together the chicken broth, aminos, tomato paste and garlic and pour over the meat mixture. Gently press the vegetables and meat so the meat is submerged in the broth mixture (this helps prevent the meat from drying out). Cook for 6 hours on low. Serve over cauliflower "rice" or soaked rice.

Teriyaki Salmon Recipe (Grain-Free, Paleo)

Teriyaki Salmon comes together in a matter of minutes!

Ingredients

For the Sauce:

• 1/3 cup fermented gluten-free tamari sauce (or coconut aminos for a Paleo option)

• 1/4 cup raw honey

• 2 tablespoons coconut vinegar

• 1 1/2 teaspoons arrowroot flour

For the Fish and Vegetables:

• 2 tablespoons coconut oil , divided

• 2 bell peppers, seeded and sliced thin

• 16 ounces wild salmon, cut into four pieces

• 5 green onions, chopped

• 1 tablespoon sesame seeds (optional)

Instructions

1. Whisk together all of the sauce ingredients in a small saucepan. Set over low heat and stir occasionally until thickened, about 5 minutes.

2. Meanwhile, heat a large sauté pan over medium heat for 2 minutes. Add 1 tablespoon coconut oil and swirl to coat. Add bell peppers to pan and cook, stirring occasionally, until spotty brown on the edges, about 5-7 minutes. Remove peppers from pan and set aside. Add remaining 1 tablespoon coconut oil to the pan and swirl to coat. Place salmon skin-side down on the skillet and let cook (without moving) until bottom is golden brown on the edges, about 3-4 minutes. Using a spatula, flip each piece of salmon over and cook (without moving) until second side is golden brown on the edges, about 3 minutes. Place each piece of salmon on a plate and drizzle with teriyaki sauce. Serve with bell peppers, cauliflower rice (if using), green onions, and sesame seeds.

Greek Salad with Beef Kabobs

Greek Salad is an iconic favorite and is so easy to make at home. I've added sirloin kebobs that have been marinated in olive oil, red wine vinegar and garlic to add some extra protein to the dish.

Ingredients

For the kabobs:

• 1 pound sirloin, cut into 1 1/2-inch cubes

• 3 tablespoons extra-virgin olive oil

• 1 tablespoon red wine vinegar

• 1/2 teaspoon garlic powder

For the salad:

• 6 ounces baby romaine

• 1/2 red onion, sliced thin

• 1/2 cup Kalamata olives

• 1/2 cup feta cheese, crumbled (omit for dairy free)

• 1/2 English cucumber, slices

- 1 pint cherry tomatoes, cut in half

For the dressing:

- 1/4 cup extra virgin olive oil

- 2 tablespoons red wine vinegar

- 2 garlic cloves, crushed

- 1/2 teaspoon Celtic sea salt

- Freshly ground black pepper

Instructions

1. Place the sirloin in a flat dish. Whisk together the olive oil, red wine vinegar and garlic in a measuring cup. Pour the marinade over the steak and lift the steak up so the marinade covers the bottom side of the steak as well. Let sit for 1 hour at room temperature, or 2-3 hours in the fridge. Heat the grill to medium (or you can use an indoor grilling pan). Thread the meat onto skewers and grill until medium-rare to medium, depending on your preference. Set aside.

2. Place the romaine, red onion, Kalamata olives and feta cheese, cucumber and tomatoes in a salad bowl. Whisk

the olive oil, red wine vinegar, garlic, and sea salt in a measuring cup. Pour the dressing over the salad. Serve the salad with the beef kabobs and season with just a bit of freshly ground black pepper.

Butter Chicken Recipe

Butter chicken is a comforting and nourishing meal that has become a family favorite these last few months. The chicken is marinated in yogurt, vindaloo spice blend, and lemon juice and then combined with caramelized onions, broth, tomatoes and cream to create a luxurious meal.

Ingredients

- For the marinade:

- 1 cup plain, whole yogurt (or coconut or almond milk yogurt for a dairy-free option)

- 1/4 cup Vindaloo spice blend

- Juice of 1 lemon

- 4 chicken breasts cut into bite-size pieces

- For the onions:

- 1 stick unsalted butter (or 4 tablespoons ghee or coconut oil for a dairy-free option)

- 2 yellow onions, thinly sliced

- 1 cup crushed tomatoes

• 1/2 cup chicken stock or broth

• 2 teaspoons Celtic sea salt

• 1/2 cup raw cream or coconut milk

• Cilantro and chopped cashews for serving (optional)

Instructions

1. Stir the yogurt, vindaloo spice blend, and lemon juice together in a medium bowl. Stir in the chicken and make sure the chicken is thoroughly coated with the marinade. Cover and place in the refrigerator to marinate for about 8-10 hours, or you can leave the mixture on the counter for 1 hour to marinate if you're short on time.

2. Melt the butter over low heat in a large sauté pan. Add the onions and cook on low heat for about 35-40 minutes, stirring occasionally until soft and caramelized. Stir in the chicken mixture (yogurt, spices and all) and increase the heat to medium. Stir in the tomatoes, stock and salt. Continue to cook, stirring frequently, until chicken is cooked through, about 15 minutes. Stir in the cream. Serve over riced cauliflower, or soaked brown rice, and top with chopped cilantro and cashews.

Slow Cooker Spaghetti S▯uash with Meatballs and Marinara (Grain-Free)

Spaghetti Squash with Meatballs is an easy slow-cooker meal that the entire family can enjoy!

You can make the meatballs with beef if you'd like, but I really like the light flavors of turkey. I tried this recipe with chicken meatballs and wasn't a fan. They were too dry after cooking for four hours in the slow cooker. One added plus – no need to make fancy meatballs, just mash the meat with an egg, salt, and pepper and they'll be good to go.

Ingredients

For the marinara:

• 2 tablespoons olive oil , plus extra for drizzling

• 1 tablespoon Italian seasoning blend

• 1 (15-ounce) jar crushed tomatoes

• 1 teaspoon Celtic sea salt , plus extra for seasoning

The squash:

• 1 spaghetti squash, cut in half and seeds removed

For the Meatballs:

• 1 pound ground organic turkey

• 1 large egg, beaten (or 2 egg yolks if you need to avoid whites)

• 1/2 teaspoon Celtic sea salt

• 1/4 teaspoon freshly ground black pepper

• Parmesan cheese for garnish (optional)

Instructions

1. Place the olive oil and Italian seasoning in a small sauce pan over medium-low heat. Heat for about 1 minute, until the herbs are fragrant, then pour into the slow cooker . Add the crushed tomatoes and 1 teaspoon sea salt and stir together.

2. Place the s□uash halves into the slow cooker, cut side up, on top of the tomato mixture. Season with sea salt and drizzle with a little olive oil.

3. In a medium bowl, combine the turkey, egg, sea salt and black pepper. Using a spoon, scoop bite-size meatballs and place into the tomato mixture.

4. Place the lid on the crock pot and cook on medium heat for 4 hours. Using a fork, remove the spaghetti squash strands from the skins and serve with meatballs and marinara. I like to throw a little parmesan on top!

When I was going through my "raw fish" cravings a few weeks ago, I made several batches of shrimp ceviche to curb the cravings.

Ingredients

• 1 pound raw wild shrimp, peeled and cut into bite-size pieces

• 1/2 cup fresh lime juice

• 1 pint cherry tomatoes, cut in half

• 1/2 cup chopped red onion

• 1/2 cup cucumber, chopped

• 1/2 cup fresh cilantro leaves, chopped

• 1 jalapeno pepper, diveined, seeded and chopped

• 1/2 teaspoon Celtic sea salt

Instructions

1. Place shrimp and lime juice in a shallow dish. Cover, and put in the refrigerator to marinate for 30 minutes.

2. Place tomatoes, red onion, cilantro, jalapeno pepper, sea salt and shrimp and lime mixture in a medium bowl. Stir until incorporated. Season to taste with salt. Serve cold.

Cream of Vegetable Soup

Cream of Vegetable Soup was one of the first recipes I tried and the entire family fell in love with this delightful soup. Abby even re🞵uested it for her birthday dinner when she turned three!

Ingredients

• 4 tablespoons butter (or 3 tablespoons duck fat for a dairy-free option)

• 2 yellow onions, chopped

• 4 carrots, chopped

• 4 large russet potatoes, chopped (or 1 large head cauliflower chopped for a lower carb option)

• 10 cups chicken stock

• 3 sprigs of fresh thyme, tied together with a piece of twine

• 4 zucchini, cut into 1-inch coins

• 2 teaspoons Celtic sea salt

• 1/2 cup raw heavy cream (or coconut milk for a dairy-free option)

• Creme fraiche, sour cream, raw shredded cheddar (optional)

Instructions

1. Melt the butter over low heat in a dutch oven . Add the onions and carrots, put the lid on the pot and let the vegetables sweat for 30 minutes. Add the potatoes and stock and increase heat to medium-high and boil. Reduce the heat to a low boil and cook until potatoes are fork tender. Add the thyme sprigs and zucchini and cook for an additional 8-10 minutes until the zucchini are tender. Remove the thyme bundle from the soup. Using a hand-immersion blender, blend the soup until smooth. Stir in salt and cream. Taste the soup and add more sea salt if needed. Ladle the soup into bowls and serve with a dollop of sour cream or creme fraiche and raw cheddar (if using).

Avocado, Mango and Pickled Onion Salad with Jalapeño Vinaigrette

If you're looking for a healthy compliment for your meals, you need to try Quick pickled onions! You can put them together in just a few minutes; after an hour, you can use them over salads, meats, vegetables and fruits.

Ingredients

For the quick pickled onions:

• 1/2 cup raw apple cider vinegar

• 1 cup filtered water

• 1 teaspoon honey

• 1 teaspoon Celtic sea salt

• 1 red onion, thinly sliced

For the Vinaigrette:

• 1/4 cup fresh lime juice

• 1/4 cup extra-virgin olive oil

• 1/2 jalapeño, seeds removed

• 1 tablespoon chopped red onion

• 1 teaspoon Celtic sea salt

For the Salad:

• 8 cups baby romaine lettuce

• 4 mangoes, cut into bite-size pieces (I prefer Champagne mangos)

• 4 avocados, cut into slices

• 1 recipe picked onions (see recipe above)

Instructions

1. Whisk the apple cider vinegar, water, honey and sea salt together in a measuring cup. Place the onions in a medium bowl and pour the vinegar mixture over the top. Let it sit for 1 hour.

2. Place the lime juice, olive oil, jalapeño, red onion and sea salt in a blender and blend until smooth. Taste and add more salt if you prefer.

3. To Serve: Place the lettuce, mangos, avocados and pickled onions in a large salad bowl (or layer it on a large platter as pictured above). Pour the dressing over the top and toss until coated. Serve immediately.

Roasted Chicken Wings (Grain-Free)

It's play-off time, which usually means lots of unhealthy snacks, but there are so many ways to make your favorites nutrient-dense and chock-full of healthy ingredients. Roasted Chicken Wings are a great substitute for the conventional variety and taste so much better!

Ingredients

• 4 pounds chicken wings

• 4 tablespoons ghee, melted (use tallow or lard for a dairy-free option)

• 2 tablespoons Herbamare

Instructions

1. Preheat the oven to 400 degrees F and adjust the rack to the middle position. Line 2 large baking sheets with unbleached parchment paper. Divide the chicken evenly between the two pans. Using a pastry brush, brush the wings with melted ghee and then season all of the wings with Herbamare.

2. Roast for 30 minutes. Using a pair of tongs, flip the wings. Roast for an additional 20-30 minutes until the

wings are golden brown on both sides. Let sit for 10 minutes, and then serve.

Conclusion

Autism, ADHD, and related mental health disorders can be challenging to manage, and it's understandable that parents of children with these conditions would want to do whatever they can to help. However, the GAPS diet requires a significant, ongoing commitment with no guarantee of success. If you're considering the GAPS diet for yourself or your child, speak with your doctor or your child's pediatrician to make certain it's the best choice for you and your family.